Operation: Life Re-Map for Divine Health - Workbook"

Companion to:
The Kingdom of God Permanent Weight Loss Principles

I0116415

www.BodyTransformationsbyTrina.com   **Trina Claiborne, Healthy Lifestyle Coach**

Published in the United States by Amazon.com
www.Amazon.com

Trina Claiborne
Operation: Life Re-Map for Divine Health - Workbook
Biblical references are New International Version (NIV)
ISBN 978-0-9988210-4-7
eISBN 978-0-9988210-5-4
Printed in the United States of America
Designed by Trina Claiborne

Also by Trina Claiborne
How I Lost 40 Pounds in 90 Days While Traveling
The Kingdom of God Permanent Weight Loss Principles

ABOUT the OPERATION: LIFE RE-MAP for DIVINE HEALTH WORKBOOK

The Operation Life Re-Map for Divine Health Workbook is a companion to The Kingdom of God Permanent Weight Loss Principles. This workbook has been designed to help you:

1. Discovery the root cause(s) of your continued weight loss battle
2. Expose you to the Kingdom of God's way to incorporate healthy lifestyle principles for divine health
3. Create your unique blueprint to remap your life in order to incorporate these principles permanently; regardless of your life complexities.

The tasks within this workbook requires 100% honesty; regardless of the painful truth. Understanding that truth often come with pain; embracing it will set you free and can take you to the next level of your desired goal(s) when taking the appropriate actions.

The BEST WAY to use the OPERATION: LIFE RE-MAP for DIVINE HEALTH WORKBOOK

The flow of this workbook is aligned with the chapters and sections in "The Kingdom of God Permanent Weight Loss Principles" book. Many of the tasks refer to the bible; therefore, have your bible handy or gain access to Bible Gateway on line at: www.Biblegateway.com for scriptural references. Although the back of the book provide room for additional notes, you may need to invest in a journal if you require more documentation space. This workbook is personal; therefore each person, family member or church member must have their own workbook.

Upon completion of this workbook, I encourage you to review it frequently to assure you stay on course according to your Life Re-Map. Keeping your eyes upon your commitment, will help ingrain your new healthy life style.

Chapter 1 Questions: The Truth about Obesity

1. After reading chapter 1:
    a. Describe your reflection in the mirror. _____

    _____
    _____
    _____

    b. List all contributing factors you honestly believe are responsible for your current reflection.

    _____
    _____
    _____
    _____
    _____
    _____

    c. How do you feel about your current reflection? _____

    _____
    _____
    _____

    d. What do you seriously want to do about your reflection? _____

    _____
    _____
    _____
    _____

Chapter 2 Question: The Dynamics of a Creator

2. According to your faith, describe your belief on how mankind came into existence & compare your beliefs to the truth as described in Genesis 1 & 2: _____

    _____
    _____
    _____
    _____
    _____
    _____
    _____
    _____

Chapter 3 Questions: Two Foundational Truths for Permanent Weight Loss

3. After mediating on III John 1: 2, list 5 other desires God designated for your life and include the scriptures that support these desires. *(To make this an easy task, go to www.Biblegateway.com an online bible where you can read or listen to the narrator, and search the scriptures using key words or phrases. You can also download the app on your smart phone at no cost.)*

   I. _____

   II. _____

   III. _____

   IV. _____

4. List 5 promises God have for your life and include the scriptures that support His promises. *(Note: Always read the scriptures in context; otherwise, you will undoubtedly miss your responsibility in the equation and not be in right standing to see the manifestation of His promises.)* Some of these promises may be repeated throughout the scriptures; but that's good news, because that's God's way of letting you know He really want those promises operating in your life.

   I. _____

   II. _____

   III. _____

   IV. _____

   V. _____

5. List 5 other scriptures that instruct **how** to guard your hearts as stated in Proverbs 4:28 (NIV) as it reads, "Above all else, guard your heart, for everything you "**do**" *(action)* flows from it."

I. _____
_____
_____

II. _____
_____
_____

III. _____
_____
_____

IV. _____
_____
_____

V. _____
_____
_____

6. Name at least five physical benefits you will reap by keeping your eyes and ears focused on God promises and His desire for your life?

a. _____
b. _____
c. _____
d. _____
e. _____

7. Explain how your words have shaped the following areas of your life *(What do you say repeatedly concerning these areas?)*:

I. **Weight Loss:**

_____
_____
_____
_____

Finance:

_____
_____
_____
_____

Marriage:

_____
_____
_____
_____

c. Reflecting upon your childhood dreams, list the dreams that have never left your heart. I refer to this as the "pre-fear stage" because I believe they are connected to your purpose in some fashion. If you have more than 3, use the notes section at the back of the book.

    i. **Childhood Dream 1**: _____

    _____

    _____

    ii. **Childhood Dream 2**: _____

    _____

    _____

    iii. **Childhood Dream 3**: _____

    _____

    _____

d. List your "natural" talents. These are things you can do with ease; whereas other may struggle to achieve your level of accomplishment. For example: Unique managerial skills, poetic skills, musician, singer, and don't forget life experiences you've overcome. The latter is a big one to list first because the negative life experiences you've overcome, and "how" you did it is your gift back to the world:

    i. **Talent 1**: _____

    ii. **Talent 2**: _____

    iii. **Talent 3**: _____

    iv. **Talent 4**: _____

    v. **Talent 5**: _____

    vi. **Life Experience** 1: _____

    _____

    _____

    vii. **Life Experience 2**: _____

    _____

    _____

e. Identify your passion(s) and explain how it/they can be used to help someone overcome struggles in that area of their life. It could be "injustice" you see happening in your community and you have resources, talents or skills to help change the situation or the outcome for others.

    i. **Passion 1**: _____

    ii. **Passion 2**: _____

    iii. **Passion 3**: _____

10. If you are operating within your life's purpose, identify how you can grow to contribute more:

a. **Growth Plan:**

_____

_____

_____

_____

_____

_____

Chapter 5: Discovering Your Purpose for Choosing to Live a Healthy Lifestyle

11. What's your main purpose or reason(s) for making the decision to live a healthy lifestyle? Ask yourself if your reason(s) is/are strong enough to keep you in the fitness game for the rest of your life? If you discover your reason(s) is/are not strong enough to promote permanent change; complete section *b. Reason Re-Map Plan below.*

   a. **Reason 1**: _____
   _____

   Reason 2: _____
   _____
   _____

   Reason 3: _____
   _____
   _____

   b. **Reason Re-Map Plan:**
   _____
   _____
   _____
   _____

Chapter 5: Discovering the Real Purpose of Food

12. Identify the food(s) you consume labeled as "your addition". It's important to determine if it's truly an addiction or a habit. An addiction is action taken "without" a trigger. Habits are action take induced by a trigger like: stressful situation/event, time of year/day or thoughts. Devise a clear plan to reverse the food abuse:

   a. **Addiction List**: _____
      i. *Addiction Re-Map Plan*:
         _____
         _____
         _____

   b. **Habit List**: _____
      Trigger(s): _____
         Bad Habit Re-Map Plan: _____
         _____
         _____

Chapters 6-8: The Function of Macro-nutrients Fats, Carbs & Protein

13. These macro-nutrients are important to include for a balance diet and the amount required differs from one person to the next. The simplest way to discover your daily dietary set-point in these areas is to partner with a healthy lifestyle coach. Self-education is another option, and if you chose this option, devise a plan to help you discovery your daily dietary set-point for each macro-nutrient. *Use the notes at the end of this workbook to document your plan.*

Chapter 9: Factors Preventing Your Weight Loss

14. Identify and devise a re-map plan for each factor preventing your fat loss goal: *(some may not apply)*

   a. **Glycogen Spillage**:

   _____
   _____
   _____

      i. *Glycogen Spillage Re-Map Plan:*

   _____
   _____
   _____

   b. **Chronic Stress:**

   _____
   _____
   _____

      i. *Chronic Stress Re-Map Plan:* _____

   _____
   _____
   _____

   c. **Loss of muscle tissue.** A body composition test will reveal muscle loss by a doctor's office for a small fee or free at your local gym.   Muscle Loss? Yes or No (circle one)

      i. *Muscle Loss Re-Map Plan:* _____

   _____
   _____

   d. **Hormonal Imbalance**:

   _____
   _____
   _____

      i. *Hormonal Imbalance Re-Map Plan:*

   _____
   _____
   _____

   e. **Lack of Exercise**: _____

   _____
   _____

      i. *Exercise Re-Map Plan:*

   _____

_____

_____

f. **Medication(s):**

_____

_____

_____

    i. *Medication Re-Map Plan:*

_____

_____

_____

g. **Lack of Water Consumption**:

_____

_____

_____

    i. *Water Consumption Re-Map Plan:* _____

_____

_____

Chapter 10: Evaluating the Fruits of Your Spirit

15. As you examine the fruits of your spirit, make two separate lists: 1st list the areas of your life you're **most proud of and why** in reference to your: career choice, daily habits, how you spend your time, how you manage your money, and the dynamics of your marital status. *(If you're not happy in these areas, see question 16.)*

    a. My Career Choice:

_____

_____

_____

_____

_____

    b. My Daily Habits & Rituals: _____

_____

_____

_____

_____

    c. How I Spend Time: _____

_____

_____

_____

_____

d. How I Manage Money: _____
_____
_____
_____
_____

e. The Dynamics of my Marriage/Family Atmosphere: _____
_____
_____
_____
_____
_____

16. List the areas of your life you're **NOT proud of and why** in reference to your: career choice, daily habits & rituals, how you spend your time, how you manage your money and the dynamics of your marital/family status. Reflect upon your answers to question # 7 above to explain how your spirit manifested the outcome of your reality in these areas.   Remember, your spirit manifest things into the natural realm through your spoken word, and your mouth speaks what's in your heart. *(Luke 6:45)* This is where you want to exam your beliefs as they are buried in your heart.

a. My Career Choice: _____
_____
_____

  • *Career Re-Map Plan:* _____
_____
_____

b. My Daily Habits & Rituals: _____
_____
_____

  • *Daily Habits & Rituals Re-Map Plan:* _____
_____
_____

c. How I Spend My Time: _____
_____
_____

  • *Time Manage Re-Map Plan:* _____
_____
_____

d. How I Manage Money: _____
_____
_____

  • *Money Management Re-Map Plan:* _____
_____
_____

e. The Dynamics of my Marriage/Family Atmosphere: _____

_____

_____

- *Marriage/Family Re-Map Plan:* _____

_____

_____

17. The final step is to devise a plan to change the outcome of your list to match the blueprint in your head. (**Note: This evaluation may require you to change your blueprint).** _____

_____

_____

_____

_____

_____

_____

_____

_____

_____

_____

Chapter 11: Starting Your Healthy Lifestyle Journey

18. Over the next 7 days, use the Appendix A: 7-Day Diet Diary to reveal your default eating patterns. It's extremely important for you to be honest with yourself, and complete it entirely according to the instructions. When completed properly, this form will reveal if you are in line with the "Daily Healthy Lifestyle Principles" listed in chapter 11. Upon your assessment, list the principles you are consistently breaking & devise a re-map plan using the notes section at the back of the workbook.
    a. Principles:
        i. _____
        ii. _____
        iii. _____
        iv. _____
        v. _____
        vi. _____
        vii. _____

Chapter 12: The Dieter's Prayer

19. I challenge you to write your personal pledge of commitment to a healthy lifestyle. I encourage you to frame it and hang it where you can look upon it every day.

    a. My Pledge to Live a Healthy Life: _____

_____

_____

_____

_____

_____

_____

_____

_____

_____

_____

_____

_____

_____

_____

_____

NOTES

Appendix A: 7-Day Diet Diary

Name: _____   Date: _____

Day 1: Wake up Time: _____
Morning Meal Time: _____
Mid-Morning Snack Time: _____
Lunch Time: _____
Afternoon Snack Time: _____
Dinner Time: _____
Night Snack Time: _____
Daily Water Intake in Ounces: _____   Other liquids: _____
# of Bowel Movements: _____
Exercise (type & duration: _____   _____
Relaxation Activity: _____
Sleep Time: ____   Describe any sleep problems: _____   _____

Please complete your 7 Day Diet Diary every day.

1. Record the time you wake up.

2. List & describe in detail ALL foods & drinks including the amounts of each. Specify in detail preparation methods like: fresh, frozen, canned, raw, cooked, baked, fried etc.

3. Record the time for EVERY meal & snack.

4. Keep track of your water intake. Please note, tea, coffee and any other liquids do not count as pure water.

5. Record the number of bowel movements per day.

6. Record any deliberate exercise activities and include the type (aerobics or resistance) and the duration.

7. Record any relaxation activities and the duration time.

8. Record the time you went to bed and include any sleep challenges experienced each day.

At the end of 7 consecutive days, compare your results with the daily healthy lifestyle principles listed in chapter 11 to determine if you're on track. To schedule a free consultation with Coach Trina, email this completed document to BodyTransformationsbyTrina@gmail.com or Fax to 678-828-5865 and log on to www.bodytransformationsbytrina.com/consultation to book the appointment.

Day 2: Wake up Time: _____

Morning Meal Time: _____

Mid-Morning Snack Time: _____

Lunch Time: _____

Afternoon Snack Time: _____

Dinner Time: _____

Night Snack Time: _____

Daily Water Intake in Ounces: _____
Other liquids:
_____
# of Bowel Movements: _____
Exercise (type & duration:
_____
_____

Relaxation Activity:
_____

Sleep Time: _____
Describe any sleep problems:
_____
_____
_____
_____
_____
_____

Day 3: Wake up Time: _____

Morning Meal Time: _____

Mid-Morning Snack Time: _____

Lunch Time: _____

Afternoon Snack Time: _____

Dinner Time: _____

Night Snack Time: _____

Daily Water Intake in Ounces: _____
Other liquids: _____
# of Bowel Movements: _____
Exercise (type & duration: _____
_____

Relaxation Activity: _____

Sleep Time: _____
Describe any sleep problems: _____
_____
_____
_____
_____

Day 4: Wake up Time: _____
Morning Meal Time: _____

Mid-Morning Snack Time: _____

Lunch Time: _____

Afternoon Snack Time: _____

Dinner Time: _____

Night Snack Time: _____

Daily Water Intake in Ounces: _____
Other liquids:

_____
# of Bowel Movements: _____
Exercise (type & duration:

_____

_____

Relaxation Activity:

_____

Sleep Time: _____
Describe any sleep problems:

_____
_____
_____
_____
_____
_____

Day 5: Wake up Time: _____
Morning Meal Time: _____

Mid-Morning Snack Time: _____

Lunch Time: _____

Afternoon Snack Time: _____

Dinner Time: _____

Night Snack Time: _____

Daily Water Intake in Ounces: _____
Other liquids: _____
# of Bowel Movements: _____
Exercise (type & duration: _____

_____

Relaxation Activity: _____

Sleep Time: _____
Describe any sleep problems: _____

_____
_____
_____
_____

Day 6: Wake up Time: _____

Morning Meal Time: _____

Mid-Morning Snack Time: _____

Lunch Time: _____

Afternoon Snack Time: _____

Dinner Time: _____

Night Snack Time: _____

Daily Water Intake in Ounces: _____
Other liquids:

_____
# of Bowel Movements: _____
Exercise (type & duration:

_____

_____

Relaxation Activity:

_____

Sleep Time: _____
Describe any sleep problems:

_____
_____
_____
_____

Day 7: Wake up Time: _____

Morning Meal Time: _____

Mid-Morning Snack Time: _____

Lunch Time: _____

Afternoon Snack Time: _____

Dinner Time: _____

Night Snack Time: _____

Daily Water Intake in Ounces: _____
Other liquids: _____
# of Bowel Movements: _____
Exercise (type & duration: _____
_____

Relaxation Activity: _____

Sleep Time: _____
Describe any sleep problems: _____
_____
_____
_____
_____

Appendix B – Sugar Name Exposure List

Although the U. S. Food & Drug Administration (FDA) requires food producers to list all ingredients in their foods, sugar can be naturally occurring (fruit or milk) or an added ingredient. Unfortunately the manufacturers are not required to expose whether the total sugar listed includes added sugar; which makes it very difficult to determine how much added sugar you're actually consuming. The best way to avoid being subjected to unwanted added sugar is to have a diet dominated by whole foods (fresh & fresh frozen foods). Below are the most common added sugar names you'll find on food labels. In addition to using this list as a resource, let your taste buds tell you the truth.

Agave Nectar
Barbados sugar
Barley Malt
Barley Malt Syrup
Beet Sugar
Brown Sugar
Buttered Syrup
Cane Juice
Cane Juice Crystals
Caramel
Carob Syrup
Castor Sugar
Coconut Palm Sugar
Coconut Sugars
Confectioner's Solids
Corn Sweetener
Corn Syrup
Corn Syrup Solids
Date Sugar
Dehydrated Cane Juice
Demerara Sugar
Dextrin

Dextrose
Diastatic Malt
Diatase
Ethyl Maltol
Evaporated Cane Juice
Free Flowing Brown Sugars
Fructose
Fruit Juice
Fruit Juice Concentrate
Galactose
Glucose
Glucose Solids
Golden Sugars
Golden Syrup
Grape Sugar
High Fructose Corn Syrup (HFCS)
Honey
Icing Sugar
Invert Sugar
Lactose
Malt
Malt Dextrin

Maltose
Malt Syrup
Mannitol
Maple Syrup
Molasses
Muscovado
Palm Sugar
Panocha
Powdered Sugar
Saccharose
Sorbitol
Sorghum Syrup
Sucrose
Sugar (granulated)
Treacle
Turbinado Sugar
Yellow Sugar
FAKE SUGARS:
   Splenda
   Aspartame

The American Heart Association (AHA) recommends no more than 9 teaspoons (38 grams) of added sugar per day for men and 6 teaspoons (25 grams) per day for women. The AHA limits for children vary depending on their age and caloric needs, but range between 3-6 teaspoons (12 - 25 grams) per day.

APPENDIX C: Understanding Food Nutrition Labels

The American Heart Association (AHA) provides education on how to read and understand food labels to help you make healthier choices. The article & diagram below were published by (AHA) on May 15, 2015 reflecting a sample food label information facts for educational purposes:

1 – Start with the serving information at the top of the label. This will tell you the size of a single serving and the total number of servings per container (package).

2 – Next, check total Calories per serving. Pay attention to the calories per serving and how many servings you're really consuming if you eat the whole package. If you double the servings you eat, you double the calories and nutrients.

The next section of information on a nutrition label is about the amounts of specific nutrients in the product.

3 – Limit these nutrients *(Saturated & Trans Fat, Cholesterol, Sodium & Carbohydrate)*: AHA recommends limiting these nutrients: Based on a 2,000 calorie diet, no more than 11-13 grams of saturated fat, as little trans-fat as possible, and no more than 1500 mg of sodium.

4- Get enough of these nutrients *(Dietary Fiber, Protein, Vitamin A &C, Calcium & Iron)*: Make sure you get enough of beneficial nutrients such as: dietary fiber, protein, calcium, iron, vitamins and other nutrients you need every day.

5 – Quick guide to % Daily Value. The % Daily Value (DV) tells you the percentage of each nutrient in a single serving, in terms of the daily recommended amount. As a guide, if you want to consume less of a nutrient (such as saturated fat or sodium), choose foods with a lower % DV – 5 percent or less. If you want to consume more of a particular nutrient like; fiber, seek foods with a higher % DV – 20 percent or more.

- Remember that the information shown in these

Nutrition Facts

Serving Size 2/3 cup (55g)
Serving Per Container About 8

Amount Per Serving	
Calories 230	Calories from Fat 72

	% Daily Value*
Total Fat 8g	**12%**
Saturated Fat 1g	**5%**
Trans Fat 0g	
Cholesterol 0mg	**0%**
Sodium 160mg	**7%**
Total Carbohydrate 37g	**12%**
Dietary Fiber 4g	**16%**
Sugars 1g	
Protein 3g	

Vitamin A	10%
Vitamin C	8%
Calcium	20%
Iron	45%

*Percent Daily Value are based on a 2,000 calorie diet. Your daily value may be higher or lower depending on your calorie needs.

	Calories	2000	2500
Total Fat	Less than	65g	80g
Sat Fat	Less than	20g	25g
Cholesterol	Less then	300mg	300mg
Sodium	Less then	2,400mg	2,400mg
Total Carbohydrate	Less then	300g	375g
Dietary Fiber		25g	30g

panels is based on 2,000 calories a day. You may need to consume less or more than 2,000 calories depending upon your age, activity level, and whether you're trying to lose, gain or maintain your weight.

- When the Nutrition Facts label says a food contains 0g of trans-fat, but includes partially hydrogenated oil in the ingredient list, it means the food contains trans-fat, but less than 0.5 grams of trans fat per serving. So eating more than one serving can exceed your daily limit of trans-fat.